THE
VEGAN CANNABIS
COOKBOOK

M000028143

*Vegan Recipes For Delicious
Marijuana-Infused Edibles*

By
Eva Hammond and Aaron Hammond
Version 2.2
Published by HMPL Publishing

Get to know your publisher at

happyhealthygreen.life

A Note from the Authors

This cookbook is the second project of mainly my wife Eva Hammond. She collected the recipes and shared some of her kitchen secrets. With my knowledge, input and experience we managed to bring you the best mouth-watering vegan cannabis edibles and recipes.

This cookbook is an essential guide for the aspiring cannabis chef. Learn how to make your vegan-proof edibles and to cook with marijuana. We bring you some modified classics from the vegan world and also include some new recipes. We start with the essential knowledge to teach you how to make and handle both edibles and cannabis-infused recipes. It all comes down to responsible use and proper know-how.

We hope that you will enjoy the information and recipes in this book and make use of the recipes that we present you!

Eva has published more books about both cannabis and vegan recipes. Aaron is well-known for his books about cannabis (marijuana) and its medical properties.

Much love and kind regards,

Eva & Aaron Hammond

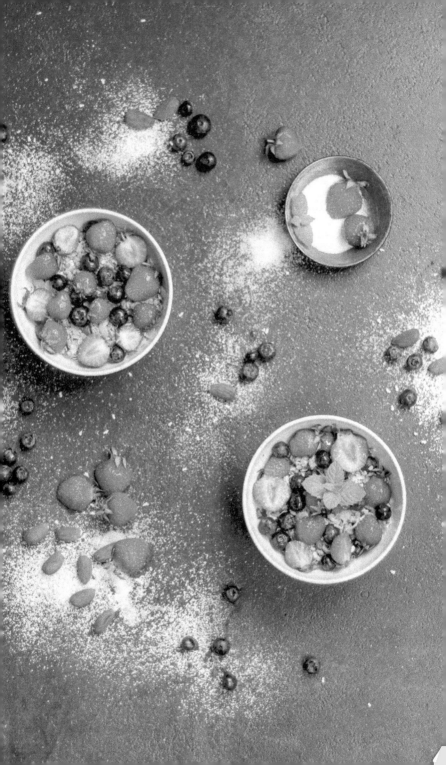

CONTENTS

ABOUT US

Welcome to the reader's circle of happyhealthygreen.life.

Subscribe to our newsletter by using this link: **http://happyhealthygreen.life/cannabis-newsletter**

And get the book 'Cannabis 101: A Short Introduction To Growing Medical Marijuana With Our Favorite Strains And Recipes For Cannabis Infused Cooking' for FREE!

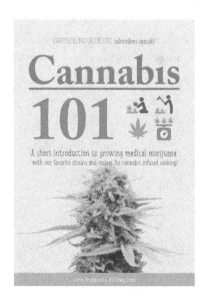

By subscribing to our newsletter, you will receive cannabis infused recipes, the best medical and recreational marijuana tips and even more free eBooks right in your inbox.

We also offer you a unique opportunity to read future cannabis books for absolutely free...

Get your hands on awesome tips, recipes and instant access to 'Cannabis 101'. Subscribe to the cannabis newsletter and grab your copy at:

http://happyhealthygreen.life/cannabis-newsletter

Enter your email address to get instant access.

* We don't like spam and understand you don't like spam either. We'll email you no more than 2 times per week.*

DISCLAIMER

The recipes provided in this report are for informational purposes only and are not intended to provide dietary advice. A medical practitioner should be consulted before making any changes in diet. Additionally, recipe cooking times may require adjustment depending on age and quality of appliances. Readers are strongly urged to take all precautions to ensure ingredients are fully cooked and safe to consume in order to avoid the dangers of food borne viruses. The recipes and suggestions provided in this book are solely the opinion(s) of the author(s). The author and publisher do not take any responsibility for any consequences that may result due to following the instructions provided in this book.

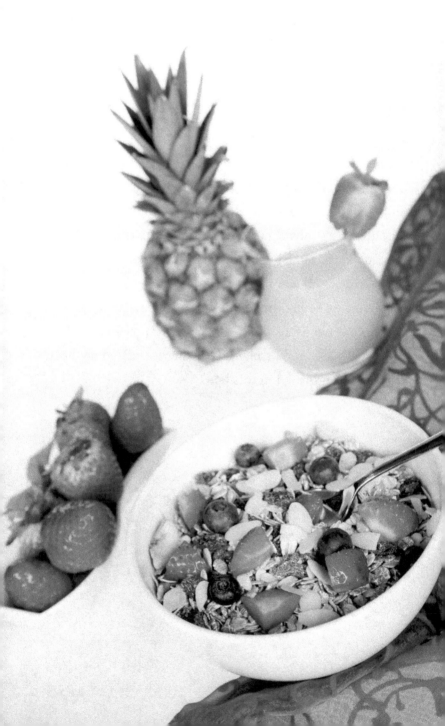

Mouth-watering Vegan Edibles

This book will bring you everything you need to know about edibles and how to make them, fitting your vegan diet.

Veganism can be a healthy lifestyle choice based on consciousness and green sustainability. If you add cannabis to the mix, you're going to have to learn some vegan infusion methods and edible recipes. This book has you covered on all the essentials, so you can start out and give these delicious organic vegan recipes a try! Topics regarding the basics about cannabis are just as important as the recipes as you're dealing with a potent medicine which can offer you great potential but also kick you in the face if you're not careful.

I mainly point at dosing your cannabis for ingestion because this is very whole different experience compared to smoking or vaporizing your bud. Simply put, the active compounds in cannabis have a stronger effect if they enter your body through your digestive system. This offers great medical potential, but what would normally be a pleasant amount when smoking, can turn your world upside down if you're inexperienced with edibles.

It cannot be stressed enough as you'll see many times throughout this book. Basic principle, smoking tolerance is definitely not the same as edible tolerance. Smoking about 200 mg of THC might be a walk in the park as a figure of speech for an experienced smoker, but if you never had a strong edible, 200mg of THC will blast you off into outer space. This could potentially be a very uncomfortable situation and it wouldn't be the first time someone ending up on IC thinking they'd overdosed on pot brownies. The author is no stranger to such effects; edibles are the choice right now but have been miscalculated in the past resulting in some unpleasant experiences. But we'll talk later about these topics when it comes to dosing, potency and reducing the potential for bad experiences.

Dosing and Measuring Your Edibles

Dosing your edibles can be super tricky but you will gain experience over time after cooking many batches of edibles. Sometimes learning will come through experience. Getting it exactly right is nearly impossible the potency can vary a lot. It might say 1000 mg on a bag of THC-infused popcorn and the bag contains a 1000 mg of THC; that doesn't mean that if you eat a piece it is always going to be the same strength and exactly the same measurements. You will notice this especially if you have a low tolerance for edibles and we will get into that in the chapter "The Right Way to Edibles. The key points to dosing your edibles are:

- Check the label before you extract if you buy it from a dispensary. Measuring without knowing your bud is a lost cause. Some producers note THC percentage on flower packaging, others note THCA. If you see a THCA percentage, use the 0.88 conversion rate to determine potential THC.

- Portion your cannabis coconut oil vertically. "Gravity impacts everything," says Davidson, "and each cannabinoid has a different molecular weight, so they will settle in different places." Oil from the bottom of the batch will be different than oil from the top, so don't scoop straight off the top.

✂ Measure carefully if you have to make single batch doses. Don't plop a big spoonful of cannabis coconut oil into the batter; get some measuring cups and fill and level them precisely.

✂ Stir well. The next thing is to stir until you're positive the batter is perfectly even and then stir some more.

✂ Portion your dough batter or other product evenly; if you did the last step you will get a more precise dosing if you measure your portion evenly.

✂ Plan the variation of potency, but be careful. If you find that your edibles are not even close in potency, I urge you to be very careful with eating more than you should initially. You could end up having an uncomfortable experience.

CALCULATING THE POTENCY OF YOUR EDIBLE

Take, for example, 100g of top-shelf Sour Diesel. Estimate the potency around approximately 20%, or about 200mg THCA per 1g of bud. This means that 200mg of THCA x 100 is 20,000mg THCA.

The conversion from THCA to THC through the process of decarboxylation is 0.88 as mentioned earlier. So this would mean that 20,000mg x 0.88 = 17,600mg maximum THC available to be decarboxylated.

Under ideal conditions, you would get a 90% efficiency of extraction in coconut oil, so that means 17,600mg x 0.9 = 15,840 mg of THC maximum to be extracted.

So with this knowledge, when your preferred dosage is 200mg per brownie, then 15,840 mg / 200 is equal to almost 80 brownies that contain around 200mg each. This is the absolute maximum; it is more likely that your brownies contain less; they could be more likely in the range of 150 to 180 mg, depending on the method and efficiency of your infusion.

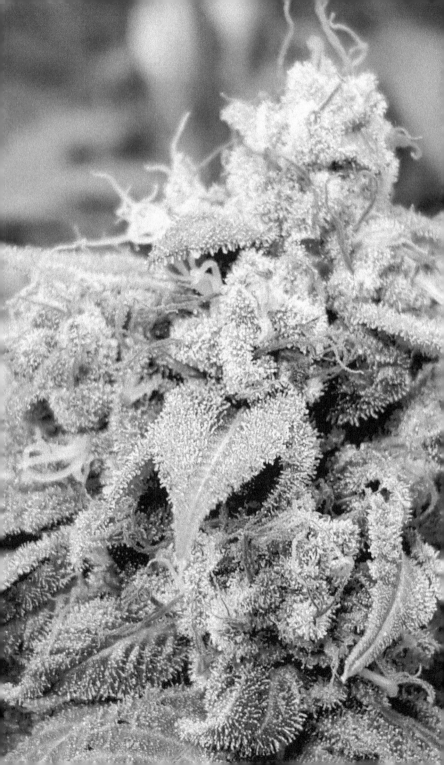

The right way to edibles is in the dosing; this can't be stressed enough. It all starts with picking the right strain for your edible when it comes to cannabis and effect. Starting with the basics for strains, there are three types; Sativa, Indica and hybrids. Hybrids are crosses between Sativa and Indica strains and are Indicated by percentage, ranging from 50/50 to 70/30 and are either Sativa or Indica dominant. Even with a 50/50 cross you can still feel the difference; for example, S5 haze is a 50/50 hybrid but has a strong and dominant uplifting Sativa effect which fades away over time into a more relaxing Indica state of mind. Even though it is classed as a 50/50 it feels Sativa dominant. This is where we get into the effects of Sativa and Indica strains.

Indica strains are known to have great medical potential and are very effective for overall pain relief and stress relief. You can benefit from Indica strains in treating insomnia and increase your appetites. Indica buds are most commonly smoked by medical marijuana patients in the late evening or even right before bed due to sleepiness and tiredness experienced when high from an Indica strain of marijuana. The most popular Indica strains currently include Bubba Kush, Blueberry and Northern Lights.

Sativa-dominant strains provide an uplifting, energetic and more cerebral high that is best suited for daytime use. A Sativa high is filled with creativity and energy as being high on Sativa can spark new ideas and creations. It offers great medical potential to patients that suffer from ADHD and COPD as well as people that benefit from cannabis in general as Sativa strains can help you get through the day without the couch-lock from indica strains.

So when it comes to edibles the effects depend on the strain but here are 5 tips that are key to a comfortable and fun edible experience.

1. Read the label or know your estimated dose

Whether buying at your local dispensary or making homemade, knowing the dosage is critical. A good dose to start with when completely new to cannabis is 5mg of THC; if you've never tried edibles but have some experience with cannabis, a good dose is 10 mg of THC; for medical use a little higher dose is acceptable depending on your condition, but the absolute maximum should be 25 mg for a first time experience.

2. Start off slow

Edibles have a different effect on your system than smoking cannabis. This is due to the fact that the THC absorbs through your stomach lining before entering your bloodstream to travel to the brain. This means that it takes more time before you feel the effects of the cannabis; it can take up to 90 minutes or more in some cases. Usually effects are felt within an hour, but don't eat more if you don't feel anything. If it is your first time, start out with a very small dose and decide after two hours whether to take more or not.

3. Keep them separate from the snacks

This is very important. Using edibles as snacks can result in consuming too much with harmful effects. Keep them put away and buy some regular snacks. This will also prevent anyone else from accidentally eating your edibles with unexpected effects.

4. Don't mix and match

The safest bet when trying edibles is to stick with one thing at a time. Even though you might feel the urge to smoke while waiting for the edible to start working, this can result in too much THC in your system at once. This goes double for using more than one edible at a time. Double dosing is for seasoned edible users only.

5. Take care of yourself

Since edibles go through the stomach, they can affect each person differently. On an empty stomach, you will be wasting edibles as your liver will break down most of the THC before it reaches your intestines. This means your edible will lose most of its effect on an empty stomach. The best thing to do is to eat a good meal at least an hour before you start on your edible.

That moment where your cannabis edible finally kicks in... It can sometimes be a scary moment if you're not prepared or if it turns out to be stronger than you had anticipated. Not to worry, thankfully Mother Nature offers us a few reset buttons if you over medicate.

- **Calm down and chill out:** Even if you just ate your whole batch of No Bake Fudge, rest assured panicking will only make it worse. Try meditation techniques paired with deep breathing exercises which will allow you to calm yourself.

- **Find a quiet and safe place:** Bright visual stimuli, loud noises and crowds can all add to the disorientation you experience during a THC high. Coupled with meditation and breathing techniques, finding a quiet place to "cool out" is one of the better ways to collect yourself.

- **Drink enough water:** "Cottonmouth" is common, and while you're medicating, the body's need for water intake increases. A nice cold glass of water will help refresh and rejuvenate, while also helping prevent severe headaches.

✂ **Eat or drink something sweet:** Cannabis has been associated with lowering or regulated blood sugar levels in the body. Eating fruits or anything with a natural sugar content will help to reduce the effects of your THC high.

✂ **Black pepper magic:** Terpenes are the wonderfully aromatic oils that plants/fruits produce naturally. These oils have natural medicinal properties that, when paired with cannabis, work together to provide a number of different effects for users. Black Pepper contains a terpene called Beta-Caryophyllene which can be used to treat anxiety or depression and also induce drowsiness. Chewing 2-3 black peppercorns can help to reduce the effects from over-medicating.

✂ **Take some CBD:** Ingesting CBD counteracts the psychoactive effects of THC by providing a sedative effect. A higher level of CBD will work to balance out the feelings associated with the THC high.

✂ **Sleep it off:** Sleeping is the most effective remedy for smoking or ingesting too much cannabis. Even though edibles take longer to digest and be processed, the grogginess you'll feel upon awakening will subside with time.

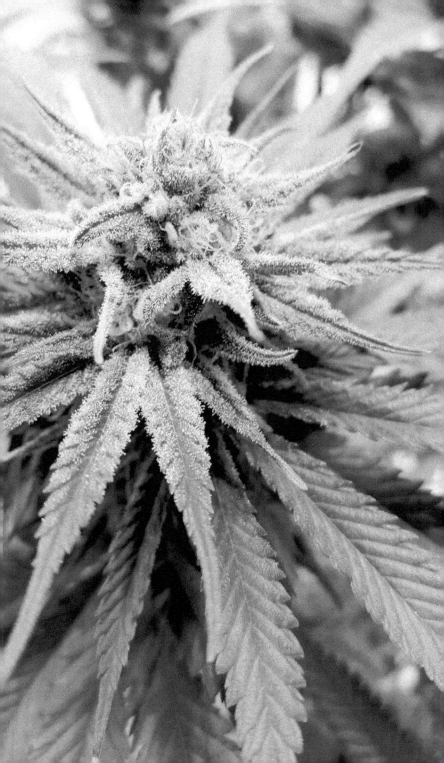

Decarboxylation is the process of turning non-psychoactive THCA into THC. To this process, all cannabinoids contained within the trichomes and resin of raw cannabis flowers have an extra carboxyl ring or group known as COOH attached to their chain. For example, THCA or tetrahydrocannabinol acid is synthesized within the trichome heads of freshly harvested cannabis flowers. In most regulated markets right now cannabis distributed in dispensaries contains labels detailing the product's cannabinoid contents. THCA, in many cases, prevails as the highest cannabinoid present in items that have not been decarboxylated such as buds or hash and certain extractions.

THCA, when consumed, has a number of known health and medicinal benefits including anti-inflammatory and neuroprotective qualities. But THCA is not psychoactive and must be converted into THC through decarboxylation before any effects can be felt.

The two main ways for decarboxylation to occur are heat and time. Drying and curing cannabis over time will cause a partial decarboxylation to occur. This is why some cannabis flowers also test for a presence of small amounts of THC along with THCA. Smoking and vaporizing will instantaneously decarboxylate cannabinoids due to the extremely high temperatures present, making them instantly available for absorption through inhalation.

While decarboxylated cannabinoids in vapor form can be easily absorbed in your lungs, edibles require these cannabinoids be present in what we consume in order for our bodies to absorb them through digestion. Heating cannabinoids at a lower temperature over time allow us to decarboxylate the cannabinoids while preserving the material so you can infuse it into your oil or butter to make edibles.

The THCA in cannabis begins to decarboxylate at approximately 220F (104.4C) after around 30-45 minutes of exposure. Full decarboxylation may require more time to occur. Choosing to decarboxylate cannabis at slightly lower temperatures for a much longer period of time will preserve terpenes. Making up for some of the characteristics in the taste of your flower, this also gives the indication that what you're eating actually tastes a bit green.

Heat and time can also cause other forms of cannabinoid degradation to occur. For example, CBN (Cannabinol) is formed through the degradation and oxidization of THC, a process that can occur alongside decarboxylation. CBN accounts for a much more sedative and less directly psychoactive experience.

In order to decarboxylate cannabis at home, all you need is some starting material, an oven set to 220-230F (104-110C) depending on your location and oven model, some parchment paper and a baking tray. Finely grind your cannabis until the material can be spread thin over the parchment and placed on your baking sheet. Allow the cannabis to bake for 45-60 minutes, or longer if you want.

Always decarb your bud before you go for infusion in oil, butter or another solvent because, even though part of that process happens though simmering your product, it has been shown that this comes nowhere close to the full potential of your material.

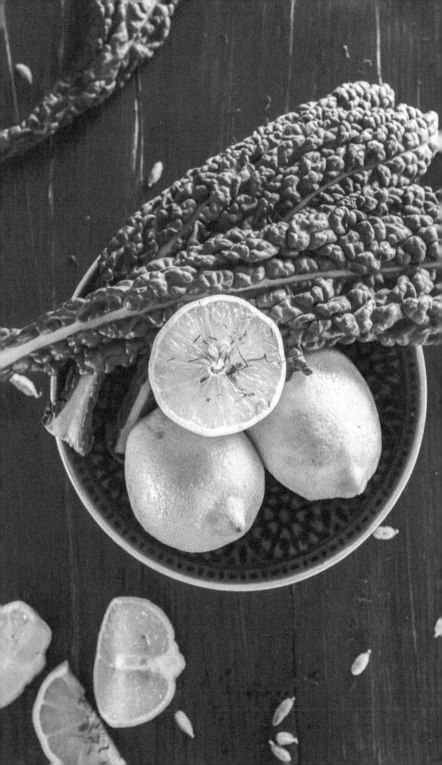

DOUBLE BOILER METHOD

When you put a pot on the stovetop, it gets hot, especially the parts of the pot that make physical contact with the heating element. For cannabis infusion this is not always the best way to go as, depending on your stove, things might get too hot too quickly. If you're using normal almond butter instead of coconut oil this can result in burning your butter in mere seconds. For coconut oil the burning point is much higher, but your oil might get too hot and lose THC as it will vaporize. The double boiler method gives the perfect opportunity to let your infusion simmer for hours around the boiling point without getting too hot too fast, and it is easier to regulate just by adding cold water in the bottom pot.

A double boiler consists of a bowl or a smaller pot placed on top of a pan of simmering water. The bowl doesn't have to touch the water but creates a seal with the bottom pan to trap the steam produced by the simmering water. The trapped steam keeps the top bowl at just about 212F (100C), the temperature at which water turns to steam, and a far lower temperature than could be achieved by putting the bowl directly on the burner. Inside the top bowl, you can melt chocolate without worrying that it will stick and burn.

You can buy a double boiler, but it's easy to make one at home. All you need is a mixing bowl (glass/Pyrex or metal) and a saucepan that the bowl will fit on top of. The two should fit tightly together; you don't want a gap between the bowl and the saucepan, nor do you want a bowl that sits precariously on a tiny saucepan. To use the double boiler, add water to the pan and bring it to a simmer, then place the bowl on top and fill it with whatever you intend to cook or melt.

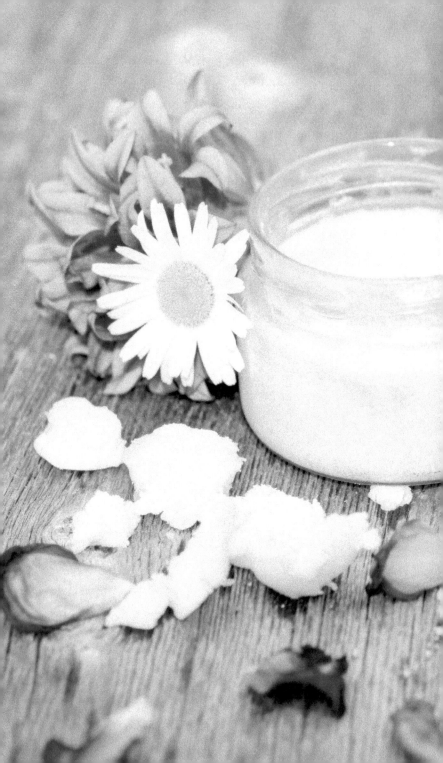

CANNABIS-INFUSED COCONUT OIL: THE BEST METHOD

What you need:

Note: Make sure you have time for this as the process can take up to 16-20 hours!

Organic Un-refined Coconut Oil:

- 1-3 Ounces of dried and decarbed cannabis
- Water
- Crockpot
- Fine metal strainer
- Coffee grinder
- Cheese cloth
- Large container
- Thermometer

Pro tip: if you want to have less of a weed scent and taste to your final product, soak your buds in water overnight

---

How to make it:

1. Grind the cannabis extremely fine. (A coffee grinder works great, but be sure not to get it too powdery. This will make it harder to strain out in the final process.)

2. In the crockpot, add the coconut oil and enough water to float the oil in the pot.
3. Set the heat on high and allow the oil to liquefy.
4. Slowly start stirring in the bud until the mixture is completely saturated. If needed, add more water.
5. Stick a thermometer in the pot with the lid closed on top, and monitor this closely it until it reaches close to 250F. Turn the crockpot heat setting to low and stir.

NOTE: Oil continues to rise in temperature after removed from heat, and takes longer to start cooling. So try to pre-emptive heat switch because this will help you keep a more accurate temperature.

6. Periodically stir the mixture and check that the temperature stays around 250 - 270 degrees.

Note: An occasional flip from low heat to hot may be needed to regulate the temp.

---

7. The mixture needs to stay below 320 degrees to avoid burning off the active ingredient. The water in the pot stops this from happening because it will evaporate first.
8. Periodically add water throughout the process to keep the cannabis submerged.
9. After 12 - 18 hours, turn off the crockpot and allow it to cool for a while.
10. Get the cheesecloth and double wrap it over your strainer. Place over a large container to catch the warm liquid.

11. Slowly pour the mixture into the cheesecloth and allow dripping. If it's not too hot, wrap the plant material and squeeze out the hot oil.

12. Continue until all the mixture has been squeezed out of the cheese cloth.

13. The remaining plant material can be saved to use for a topical compress, although most of the medicinal properties lie within the oil still trapped in the spent bud.

14. Put the container of hot oil/water in the fridge overnight and allow the oil to rise to the top.

15. The water that was added during the process catches all the extra plant material and brown carcinogens from the mixture. This allows for a much cleaner tasting product.

16. Pop the hardened green coconut oil off the top and discard of the water.

17. You are now left with a green chunk of coconut oil that is ready to use for the recipe of your liking.

18. Store in the fridge until ready to use. Allow to warm before adding to recipes.

Pro Tip: Coconut oil is a good substitute for most baking. It can replace butter in many recipes and some people like to add it to a hot beverage for an easy medication.

COCONUT OIL INFUSION METHOD: THE QUICK METHOD

What you need:

- ◆ Coconut oil – organic, un-refined
- ◆ 1 oz. of cannabis flower or trim (you can use less if you like)
- ◆ Spatula
- ◆ Strainer – fine metal
- ◆ Double boiler
- ◆ Grinder (coffee grinder)
- ◆ Cheesecloth
- ◆ Jar for storage
- ◆ Jar or a bowl where the metal strainer can fit

How to make it:

1. Always make sure that the buds you are using are decarbed.
2. Also, make sure you use 1 oz. or fewer buds for this recipe as greater amounts would require a longer cooking process and the results wouldn't be the same.
3. To get started, grind your buds, but not too finely – grind it into bigger pieces, but not chunks.
4. The ratio for this recipe would be 1:10, which would be 1 oz. of buds and 10 oz. of oil. Take the double boiler, put it on the stove and set up the stove on low heat. Pour coconut oil into the double boiler.

5. The oil needs to be completely melted so you will need to stir it. Use a spatula for stirring – this way the oil will melt a lot faster.

6. When the oil is melted and slowly simmering, being heated up to perfection where you can smell it, it is time to add the bud you have previously ground. Add it to the oil and stir it well, so all the pieces are coated with oil.

7. Now, let the buds simmer together with the oil until the temperature of 220F is reached. This is a perfect temperature for simmering cannabis buds.

8. This process of simmering should last somewhere between 1 and 2 hours; you will have to occasionally stir the mixture every 5 to 10 minutes.

9. The oil with buds will look brownish and burnt and should have a scent of coconut butter and popcorn. That is the way it is supposed to look and smell, so no worries there.

10. After 2 hours, turn the heat off and remove the boiler from the stove. Let the oil cool off slowly without rushing the process.

11. Before you begin the process of straining, you can leave the pot with the oil in the fridge overnight to increase the potency of your mixture.

12. The next step is straining. Put the cheesecloth on the strainer and place the strainer in the jar/bowl you chose to fit the strainer. Now pour the oil through the strainer, pouring it slowly.

13. Use the lidded jar or a similar container for keeping the oil stored.

14. You can use the oil right away after it has been prepared and cooled or you can use it later. Keep the oil stored in the fridge. This oil will work perfectly for baking cakes, brownies and cookies.

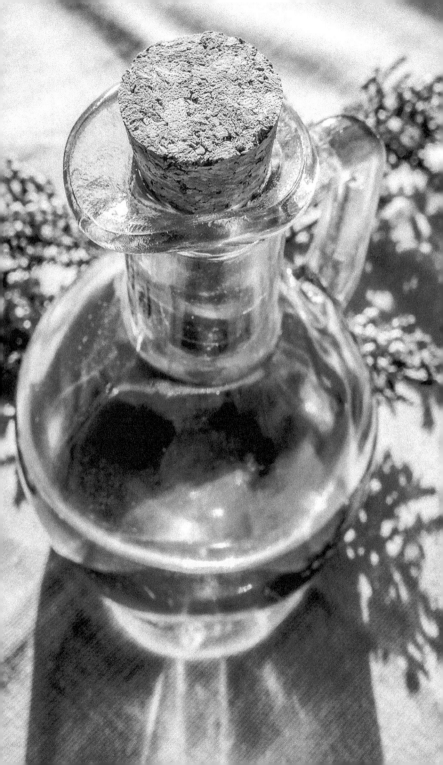

CANNA-OIL INFUSION METHOD

What you need:

- 1 oz. of cannabis buds or leaves (decarbed and ground into smaller pieces, but not too finely ground.)
- 1 oz. of Olive oil

Note: We use less olive oil, forgetting about the 1:10 proportion here as olive oil has a 25% infusion rate, unlike coconut oil that has a 90% infusion rate. That is why we use less cannabis for the coconut oil infusion method.

- Double boiler, saucepan or a pot of your choice (we recommend beginners use a double boiler rather than a saucepan or pot.)
- Cheesecloth and strainer
- Grinder
- Spatula

How to make it:

1. Make sure that buds and/or leaves you are using have been through decarboxylation process before you use them for olive oil infusion method.
2. First grind the buds into smaller pieces by using a grinder – you can use a coffee grinder without any problem or go for any type of grinder you might have.

3. Put double boiler on the stove and put the stove on low heat.

4. Pour the oil into the boiler and heat on low.

5. When the oil has heated and you can smell it that means it is time to gradually add the cannabis buds you have.

6. Stir it all well until all of the cannabis is coated in oil. When the temperature has reached 220F to 245F maximum – not more than that or you will "fry up" the THC and destroy a perfectly good cannabis – you should let the oil simmer for about 40 minutes, occasionally stirring every 5 minutes. Remember to keep the heat on low.

7. After the 40-minute simmer is over, remove the pan/double boiler from the stove and let it cool.

8. After the oil is cooled, use strainer and cheesecloth for straining.

9. Keep the oil in the seal protected jar or in an airtight container.

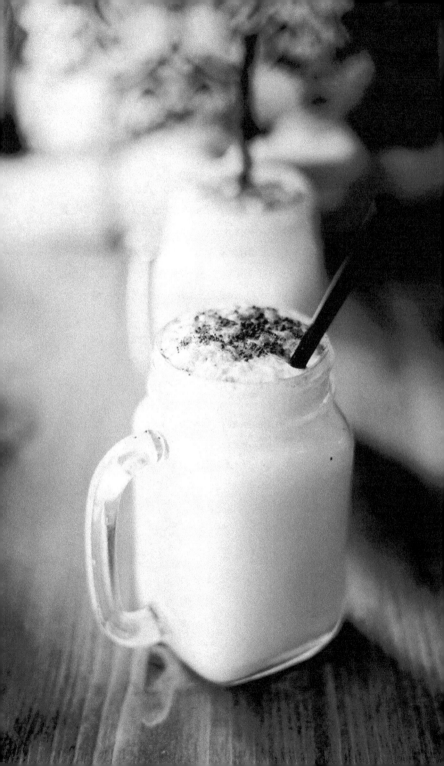

ALMOND MILK INFUSION METHOD

What you need:

- ◆ 1 pack of almond milk
- ◆ 1 oz. of cannabis buds (buds need to be finely ground, almost into dust: add one
- ◆ thumb of cannabis for each one-quarter of milk. The more milk you use, the more
- ◆ cannabis that must be added to fit the proportion.)
- ◆ Double boiler or a pot/pan
- ◆ Spatula

How to make it:

1. Pour the amount of milk you want to use for making cannabis almond milk directly into the double boiler or in the pot if you choose. Bring it to a simmer on low heat.
2. Add cannabis to the milk after it starts to simmer, gradually adding ground buds bit by bit until the buds are all covered in milk.
3. Let the milk with cannabis simmer for about 40 minutes while occasionally stirring .
4. Use cheesecloth, strain thoroughly to make sure every bit of green milk is strained.
5. Let the milk cool for a while. You can serve it in small glasses for shots or you can drink it to fit your taste, either warm or completely cool.

6. The milk is best consumed in the next 2 days. It should be kept in the fridge no longer than 2 days and stored in a sealed container to prevent spilling and spoiling.

7. In case you would like to make bigger batches of almond cannabis milk, you can keep it frozen for longer than two days then thaw before being consumed.

8. If a skin appears on top of the milk, this is perfectly normal – you just need to stir the milk a bit and the skin will break.

VEGAN CANNABIS RECIPES

Now that you have learned everything you need to know about cannabis edibles, infusion methods and the crucial process of decarboxylation that turns THCA into THC, you are ready to start making your very first cannabis infused snacks and sweets. Here are 20 recipes for the perfect cannabis infused vegan edibles.

Let's get started!

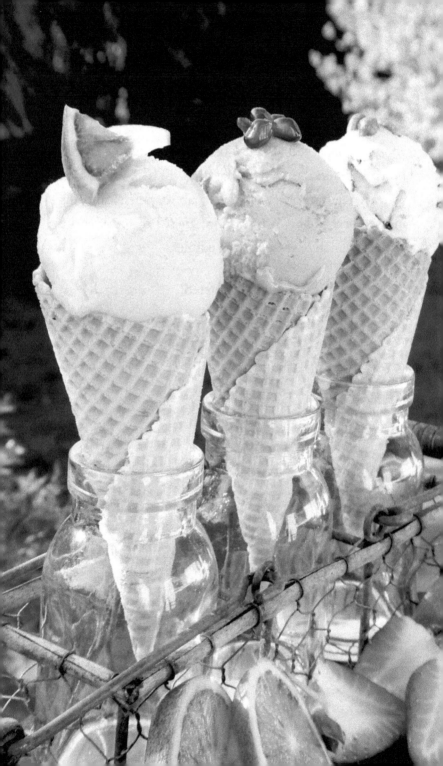

RECIPE #1: ALMOND AND BANANA INFUSED ICE CREAM

Almond and Banana Ice Cream and with Cannabis? Heaven on earth, especially during long, hot summer days!

You will need coconut oil infused with cannabis for this recipe. The amount given below is set for 4 servings of ice cream. If you are making bigger batches, be sure you increase the amount of cannabis infused oil.

What you need:

- ½ cup of coconut oil infused with cannabis
- 3 medium sized, sliced bananas (frozen)
- 1 cup of coconut cream
- ½ teaspoon of almond extract (alternatively you can use vanilla extract)
- 2 tbsp. of maple syrup – pure
- 1/3 cup of coconut flakes (you can also use coconut shreds)
- 1/3 cup of sliced almonds (you can also use chopped, unsalted)
- 1/3 cup of vegan chocolate chips

How to make it:

1. Use a blender for blending bananas until they become crumbs. After bananas are blended, add the extract of your choice, vanilla or almond, maple syrup and coconut cream. Mix them all together with blended bananas until smooth.

2. Use from 2 to 4 pulses to blend chocolate chips, almonds and coconut shreds into the mixture. After the last pulse, add coconut oil infused with cannabis. Another pulse and you are done!

3. Keep the ice cream in a sealed container placed in the freezer. You can serve it right away if you like your ice cream mildly cool and soft or you can freeze it and eat it later.

Recipe #2: Cannabis Oatmeal Bars with Peanut Chocolate

Want to grab a tasty, sweet, flavorful oatmeal bar? No fuss! This simple recipe has only a couple of ingredients you probably already have.

What you need:

- 1 cup of peanut butter –unsalted, all natural peanut butter
- ½ cup of infused coconut oil
- 2 ¼ tbsp. of maple syrup – pure, all natural
- 1 ¼ cups of oats - use the one that's gluten-free

Topping:

- ½ cup of chocolate chips (use the vegan version)
- 1 tbsp. and ¼ cup of peanut butter (unsalted, all natural)

How to make it:

1. Get your infused coconut oil ready along with a baking tray with wax or baking paper.
2. Take a double boiler and heat it on low. Add maple syrup and peanut butter, mixing those together. Add almond oil infused with decarb cannabis and stir, letting it all warm up in the boiler, and simmer for

about 20 minutes. You will notice bubbles being created as the mixture is slowly being heated up.

3. When the mixture is heated up and finely melted, you need to add the oats you have set aside for making oatmeal bars. Stir it well until combined in one smooth mixture.

4. Pour the mixture into the baking pan, using a spatula so that the mixture you are pouring is evenly layered across the baking tray.

5. You will need the double boiler again to make the topping for your bars. Add the chocolate chips and peanut butter you have set aside for the topping and stir until melted and smooth.

6. Use melted chocolate to top the oatmeal mixture layered in the baking tray.

7. Leave in the fridge to cool or put in the freezer for 40 minutes if you want to cut out genuine oatmeal bars. Serve and enjoy!

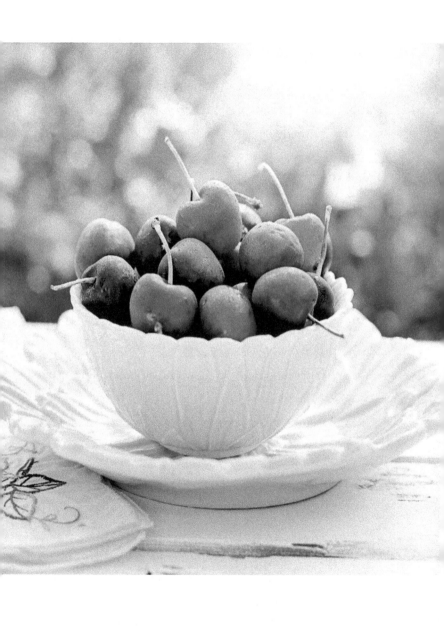

RECIPE #3: CANNABIS CHERRY CHOCOLATE BITES

We have a tasty triple C in this recipe with a wonderful combination of Chocolate, Cherry and Cannabis. Let's see how it's made.

What you need:

- Coconut oil infused with cannabis (see previous recipe)
- ¾ cup of almond butter
- ¼ cup of maple syrup, again use pure, all natural
- ½ cup of cherries, dried and chopped
- ¾ cup of coconut (shredded or coconut flakes, preferably sugar-free)
- 2 tbsp. of flaxseed (alternatively, use ground chia seeds)
- ½ cup of oats – gluten-free
- 2 tbsp. of cocoa powder – sugar-free
- ¼ cup of chocolate chips - vegan

How to make it:

1. First mix all dry ingredients and pour them all in a single bowl.
2. Add maple syrup and almond butter to the dry mixture, fold and stir with a spatula until you have made a smooth, well-combined mixture.
3. Scoop some of the mixture into your hands. Roll it up

and press with palms making the mixture into bites. You can add more dried cherries and chocolate chips by pressing them into the bites.

Recipe #4: No Bake Cannabis Brownie Bites

This is a tasty classic wrapped in new light with this baked delight. And the best thing - it's simple to make and even easier to enjoy!

What you need:

- 3 tbsp. of cannabis infused almond milk (see previous recipe)
- 2 tbsp. of nut butter (or seed butter)
- ¼ cup of coconut flour
- 4 tbsp. of brown rice syrup
- ¼ cup of cocoa powder – sugar-free
- ½ cup of chocolate powder (enrich with vegan protein powder)

How to make it:

1. Be sure that you have canna-milk prepared before you make this recipe. You can prepare it 1 or 2 days in advance or have it frozen, or you can make it just before you decide to try this recipe.
2. This recipe is fairly simple because you just need to put all the ingredients into the food processor or in a blender, blending them all together. The mixture you are looking for should be smooth and not too sticky. You can add more canna-milk or more coconut flour

if needed for the mixture to look smooth without being sticky.

3. The only thing left to do is to scoop some of the mixture into your hands – you will be making balls out of the mixture, placing them in a bowl or in a tray. You can keep brownie bites at room temperature or, if you want to keep them fresh for an extended period of time, you can place them in an airtight container and store in the fridge.

RECIPE #5: DANK SNICKERS

Believe it or not, you can now have cannabis enriched snickers. Snickers is tasty and delicious by itself, just imagine the explosion of tastes once you try this vegan version starring cannabis buds.

What you need:

- ¼ cup of peanuts – whole, unsalted
- 1/3 cup of chocolate chips – small, vegan
- 1/3 cup of coconut oil infused with cannabis (see previous recipe)
- 6 pitted Medjool dates
- 2 tbsp. water
- ¼ tsp. of vanilla extract
- Pinch of salt

How to make it:

1. This amount is set for 6 snickers bars. If you want to make bigger batches increase the amount of ingredients accordingly. First take a blender or food processor and blend water, dates, vanilla extract and a pinch of salt. Pulse until the mixture is smooth.
2. Pour oil and chocolate into the double boiler. Melt the chocolate with oil on low heat for about 20 minutes stirring occasionally until the chocolate is smooth and melted.

3. You will now need molds as you will take one teaspoon of the melted chocolate and pour it into the molds. Let the chocolate cool in the freezer until hard.

4. Once the chocolate in the molds is hardened, you will take 5 to 6 pieces of peanuts and put them in the molds with the chocolate.

5. Next, you will take the date paste you have blended in the food processor and pour some over the peanuts in each mold. Take the remaining chocolate and pour it over date caramel paste and peanuts.

6. Place the bars back into the fridge until hardened.

7. You can also keep the bars in a plastic sealed bag where they can stay fresh for a couple of weeks if kept in the freezer.

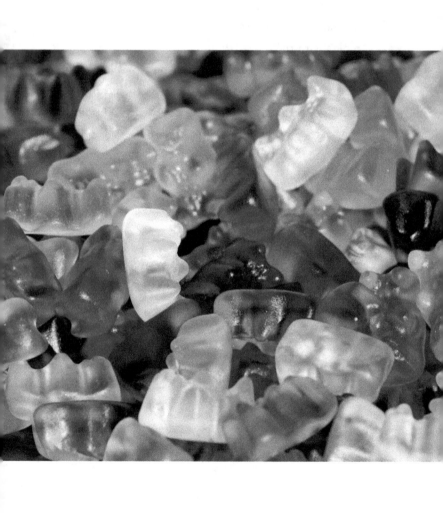

RECIPE #6: MEDICATED FRUIT GUMMIES

Yummy, gummy. If you like gummy bears, you will love this. You can make gummy candy at home and have it enriched with cannabis!

You can create a couple of batches with different flavors: for each batch, use 1 cup of berry juice/orange juice/beet juice/strawberry juice or whichever flavor comes to mind.

What you need:

For orange juice:

- ◆ Use 1 tbsp. of maple syrup and 1 tbsp. of coconut oil infused with cannabis (see previous recipe)

For other flavors:

- ◆ Use ¼ cup of berry jam combined with 1 tbsp. of coconut oil infused with cannabis (see previous recipe)
- ◆ 1/2 teaspoon of agar powder

How to make it:

1. For orange juice gummy candy, in a pan mix the syrup, oil and agar powder. For berry juice/beet juice/strawberry juice, mix the juice, agar powder, the jam

and oil in food processor or blender and blend until the mixture is smooth.

2. When preparing orange juice candy, bring the mixture to a simmer then remove it and let sit for 5 minutes. For berry candy, pour into another pan and bring it to a simmer after being blended. Let the mixture rest for 5 minutes as well.

3. Pour the mixtures you have in separate molds – you can choose any shape you like or just pour the mixture into shallow containers.

4. Place the molds with the mixtures in the fridge and let the candy rest there for 3 hours.

5. You can coat the candy with sugar and keep them in the fridge if there are leftovers.

RECIPE #7: CANNABIS AND
CASHEW CARAMELS

These caramels are pretty tasty and healthy as well. What is even better is that they are even simple to make. You will need two separate grocery lists – one for the caramel and the other for caramel clusters.

What you need:

For Caramel:

- 2 cups of dates – pitted
- ¼ tsp. of salt – grain, sea salt
- ¾ cup of water – you will need hot water
- 2 tsp. of vanilla extract – pure

For Caramel Clusters:

- Caramel (make it yourself)
- 1 cup of chopped cashews with a pinch of salt
- 1 1/2 cups of chocolate chips – vegan
- 1 tbsp. of coconut oil infused with cannabis

How to make it:

1. Start by making the caramel. Take the dates you have pitted and put them in the hot water. It would be best to put them in boiling water so the dates become

softer. Leave them in the water for 1 or 2 hours or at least until they are soft enough.

2. Then take the dates and the water that remain from boiling and put them together in the food processor. Pulse until you get a creamy and partially sticky cream.

3. Once the cream is looking nice and smooth, take the vanilla extract and a pinch of salt and pulse again until combined and smooth.

4. Now that you have the caramel, you will start with making clusters. First, toast the cashews in a skillet until they turn brownish.

5. Next, melt the chocolate in the double boiler. As you are melting the chocolate, add the oil infused with cannabis, stir and cook on low heat until the chocolate is melted and smooth, well combined with the cannabis-infused oil.

6. Use a spoon to take bits of cashews and put them on a baking tray, one by one. You should have about twenty scoops.

7. Now it's time to use the caramel you made. With a spoon, scoop a bit of caramel to top the cashews and bring them together.

8. Take the melted chocolate and pour it over the cashews with caramel.

9. Put the tray in the fridge for the caramels to harden and for the chocolate to form a shell. If you want to keep your leftovers, keep them in a sealed container. You can keep them in the fridge for a week, or put them in the freezer and keep them for two weeks.

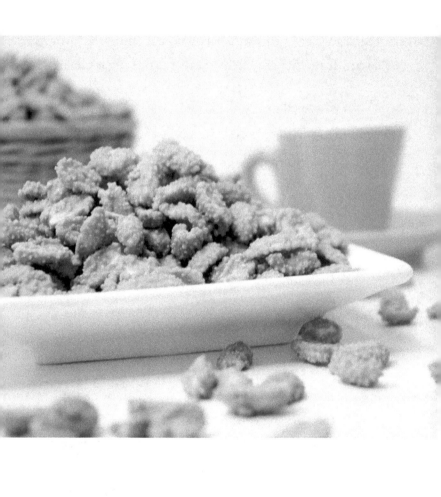

Recipe #8: Cannabis Chocolate Fudge

I bet you love chocolate fudge! Well, who doesn't, right? Here is a vegan pro-cannabis version of one of the favorite sweet treats that are likely to satisfy your sugar cravings.

What you need:

- 3 tbsp. of coconut oil infused with cannabis (see previous recipe)
- ¼ cup of coconut butter – not melted
- 1 tsp. of vanilla extract
- ¾ cup of cocoa powder
- ¼ cup of maple syrup or brown rice syrup
- Pinch of salt

How to make it:

1. Place all ingredients except for the syrup in a double boiler. Save the syrup for the end so it doesn't stick due to heat. Turn the stove to low heat and stir so that the ingredients don't stick to the bowl of the double boiler. Add the syrup at the end when the mixture becomes smooth and all ingredients are well combined. Don't allow the ingredients to get too hot; if you notice that the boiler is getting too hot, remove

it from the stove, cool it a bit then put back on. Repeat as necessary until done.

2. Once there are no lumps and the mixture is smooth, add the syrup and stir. Add the salt. Taste the mixture to see if you need more salt as this ingredient helps the chocolate in the fudge stand out.

3. Pour the mixture into the cupcake molds with cupcake paper. Put in the fridge to cool and harden. You can keep them in the fridge for a week.

Recipe #9: Raspberry and Chocolate Cannabis Candy

If you like raspberries, you will love this raspberry candy – it's creamy and crunchy at the same time and deliciously sweet, but also healthy!

What you need:

- ¾ cup of cashews, raw –soaked and drained
- 1 can of coconut cream – small pack
- 1 tsp. of lemon juice – freshly squeezed
- ¼ cup of maple syrup or brown rice syrup – pure
- 2 cups of chocolate chips – vegan version
- 2 tbsp. of coconut oil infused with cannabis
- Pinch of salt
- 5 oz. of raspberries – drained and thawed

How to make it:

1. Put the cashews in the blender or a food processor and blend until smooth and turned into paste – it's better if you keep the cashews soaked in water overnight to soften them.

2. Once you have made the paste out of cashews, put the rest of the ingredients except the chocolate and coconut oil infused with cannabis in the food

processor. Pulse until you have a smooth and creamy paste.

3. Next take the double boiler and melt the chocolate by adding chocolate chips and coconut oil infused with decarb cannabis. Melt on low heat and stir until the chocolate is completely melted and smooth.

4. You will now make filled candy; take some chocolate with a spoon and spread it over molds of your choice so every inch of the molds is covered with melted chocolate. Put it in the freezer for the chocolate to freeze and harden.

5. Once the chocolate molds are ready take some of the raspberry cream and place it in the chocolate covered molds.

6. Next, top the molds with the remaining chocolate so that the raspberry cream is all covered, and the cream is all packed and wrapped in chocolate. Return the molds to the fridge and keep the candy in there until hardened and cool.

RECIPE #10: COCONUT AND CANNABIS LEMON TART

This recipe can't possibly sound more refreshing, especially if you have a sweet tooth and need something tasty, sweet and healthy to lift your spirit.

What you need:

You will need two separate grocery lists, one for the crust and the other for the filling.

Crust:

- ½ cup of almonds
- ½ cup of pecans
- ½ cup of dates
- ½ cup of unsweetened coconut flakes (leave some extra for sprinkling)

Filling:

- 8.5 oz. of coconut cream – canned
- 1 ½ freshly squeezed lemon – juice
- ½ cup maple syrup
- 2 tbsp. of coconut oil infused with cannabis
- 1 tsp. of lemon zest
- ½ tsp. of agar powder
- 2 tbsp. of cornstarch

◆ ¼ cup of starch powder

How to make it:

1. First, take all the ingredients you have prepared for making a crust and put them in the food processor. Pulse it until the mixture is well blended.

2. In a pie pan sprinkle some coconut flakes evenly then press the crust mixture until you have a base for your tart. Place the dish with the base in the fridge and leave it there until you have finished preparing the filling for the tart.

3. Mix coconut oil infused with cannabis, coconut cream, lemon juice, lemon zest, agar powder and the syrup together in a saucepan on low heat, whisking the mixture until it starts to simmer. Remove from the stove and mix the starch with water until starch is dissolved and well mixed with water, then add to the mixture.

4. Put the saucepan back on the stove and whisk mixture on medium heat until it turns thick. It should take about 10 minutes.

5. When the mixture is thick and ready, allow it to cool, then pour it over the tart base you have previously made. Return the dish to the fridge for at least 2 hours before serving.

RECIPE #11: CANNABIS AND COCONUT CHEESECAKE WITH LIME AND AVOCADO

Lots of tasty and exotic ingredients in this recipe will satisfy your hunger for something sweet and healthy, of course with cannabis infused oil as the main star.

What you need:

You will need two separate grocery lists, one for the first layer and one for the second layer of the cheesecake.

First layer:

- ¾ cup of dates – pitted and soaked in the water so the dates are softened
- 1 cup of mixture: hazelnuts, brazil nuts and almonds

NOTE: you can mix other nuts if you prefer a different combination.

- 2 tablespoons of canna-milk: you can prepare canna-milk in advance by following our recipe

Second layer:

- 1 cup of cashews – soaked

- 1 tbsp. of chia seeds

- 1 cup of coconut oil infused with cannabis
- 1/2 cup of agave
- One lime - pulp and lime juice
- 1 avocado – medium, ripe
- ½ cup of coconut flakes

Sprinkling and garnish:

- 1/3 cup of coconut flakes
- 3 cups of sliced strawberries

How to make it:

1. Making the first layer for the cheesecake is fairly simple as you only need to put the nut mixture into the blender and pulse until you get a flour-like mixture. Then pour the canna-milk in the blender along with the soaked dates (without the water you used for soaking) and pulse until smooth. Stop pulsing to scrape the mixture off the sides and pulse some more until you have dough.

2. Place the dough on a baking tray or any tray you use for baking pies and place it in the fridge until you make the second layer. It can stay in the fridge for a bit longer if needed for the dough to cool.

3. For the second layer, take the coconut oil and melt it in a pot on low heat. Once that is ready, take the cashews and oil and pour in the blender – blend well with chia gel, avocado, lime pulp, lime juice and agave. Pulse until you have a smooth paste.

4. Next, stir the mixture a bit and pour it over the first layer spreading it evenly. Put the cheesecake in the freezer and keep it there for a couple of hours.

5. Garnish with strawberries and coconut flakes or shreds.

RECIPE #12: CANNABIS AND CARROT BALLS

This is a fine version of classic carrot cake – no bake and enriched with proteins and cannabis.

What you need:

- ¾ cup of oats
- ½ cup of dates
- 1 cup of cashews – raw
- 4 oz. of applesauce – unsweetened and mixed with coconut cannabis oil
- 35 g of vanilla vegan protein powder
- 1/2 teaspoon of cinnamon dust
- ¼ teaspoon of nutmeg
- 1 grated carrot – large
- 1/8 teaspoon of cloves
- 1/2 cup of chopped walnuts
- 1/3 cup of coconut - unsweetened

How to make it:

Whisk the cannabis infused coconut oil with the applesauce before using it in the recipe.

1. To the food processor add applesauce, cashews, dates, protein powder, oats and all the spices. Pulse

until completely mixed and turned into a dough-like mixture.

2. Next add the carrots and walnuts and blend. Pulse until you have a slightly sticky dough.

3. Take the coconut flakes or shreds and put them in a bowl.

4. Make little balls out of the dough and roll them in the coconut flakes, placing them on a tray.

5. Place the tray in the fridge and cool the balls for 30 minutes before serving. You can keep the leftovers fresh in a sealable container.

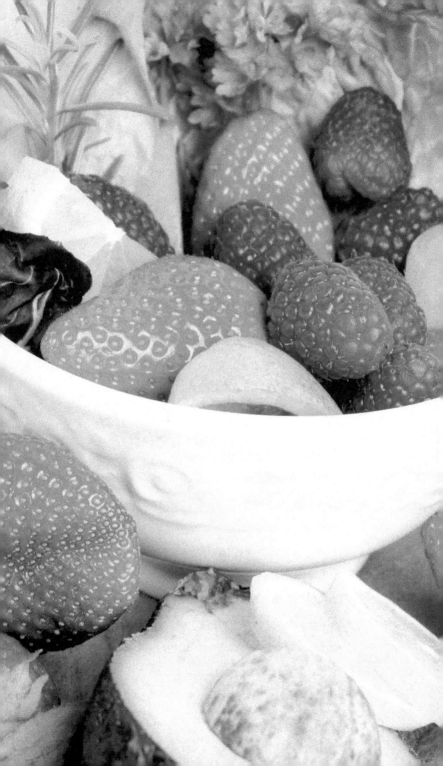

Recipe #13: Apricot and Cannabis Bites

This protein and fiber rich low-calorie desert with cannabis and apricot as the main stars will surely let you indulge in enjoyment!

What you need:

- 2 tbsp. of coconut oil infused with cannabis
- 1 cup of almonds
- 1 cup of raisins
- 10 chopped and dried apricots
- 1/2 teaspoon of cinnamon powder
- 1/2 cup of coconut shreds – sugar-free

How to make it:

- First, place almonds, cinnamon, coconut oil and raisins in a blender or food processor and pulse until you have a smooth paste. This won't take more than a couple of minutes.
- Next, add apricots to the blender and pulse for half a minute. Then, add the coconut shreds and pulse for a couple of more seconds.
- Take plastic wrap and put the dough on it pressing it into a square. Next, wrap it up entirely in the plastic wrap and place it in the fridge.

- Keep it in the fridge for half an hour then take it out and cut it in equal small squares.
- Keep the leftovers in a sealable container to keep the bites fresh.

RECIPE #14: CANNABIS AND MANGO ICE CREAM

This is the simplest recipe and probably the most refreshing one, too. Try it out and enjoy the smooth taste and refreshing flavor of mango, empowered by cannabis.

The amount of ingredients is for a single serving – increase the amount of ingredients if you want to make more servings.

What you need:

- 1 cup of mango – frozen and chopped
- 2 peeled frozen bananas
- 1 tbsp. of coconut oil infused with cannabis
- For garnish, have some grated dark chocolate

How to make it:

1. Slice the bananas. Put bananas and mango in a blender with coconut oil. Blend until you have a smooth mixture.
2. You can freeze the ice cream or eat it immediately if you like your ice cream soft and mildly cold. Top it with dark chocolate.

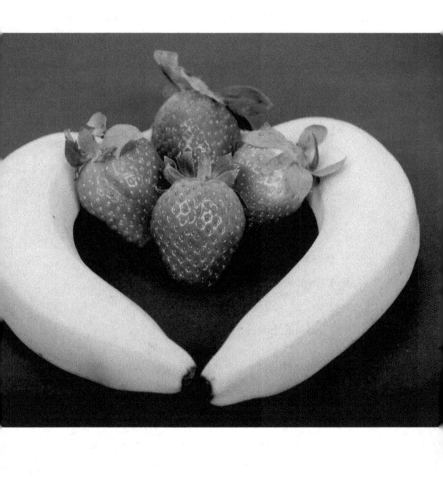

Recipe #15: Single Bowl Banana Bread with Cannabis

Banana bread is an extremely delicious classic, but this single serving banana bread with cannabis will blow your mind.

What you need:

- 1 teaspoon of coconut oil infused with cannabis
- ½ banana
- 2 tbsp. of flour – whole wheat
- 1/8 teaspoon of baking powder
- 1/4 teaspoon of cinnamon dust
- ½ teaspoon of vanilla extract
- 1 tbsp. of sugar – organic
- 1 tsp. of walnuts
- Pinch of chocolate chips - vegan

How to make it:

1. Start by mashing the banana in a bowl, adding all ingredients from the list except walnuts and chocolate. Mash until the mixture you are making is smooth.
2. Add chocolate chips and walnuts. Spray the bowl of the double boiler and pour the mixture into the bowl.
3. Warm the mixture up, cooking on low heat for one and a half minutes, but be careful not to overcook it. Let it cool for a bit and enjoy.

RECIPE #16: ALMOND MILK CHOCOLATE PUDDING WITH AVOCADO

This is an amazingly easy and yet marvelously tasty recipe for chocolate pudding – dairy-free and pro-cannabis.

What you need:

- 1/2 cup of cannabis-infused almond milk (see previous recipe)
- 1 avocado – ripe
- ¼ cup agave
- ½ cup of cocoa – unsweetened
- ½ teaspoon of vanilla extract

How to make it:

1. Make sure you have made canna-milk in advance or just before trying this recipe out. Also, make sure that the cannabis used for making canna-milk is decarb.
2. Combine canna-milk and stevia/agave in a double boiler on low heat until the mixture is smooth and agave is dissolved. Give the mixture some time to cool.
3. Remove the pit and the skin from the avocado and put it in the blender along with the cocoa powder and vanilla extract. Pulse until blended to form a smooth mixture.

4. Mix canna-milk and stevia mixture with avocado and cocoa mixture and blend some more until you have a smooth mixture with all ingredients combined.
5. Pour into bowls and put in the fridge to cool. Serve with berries.

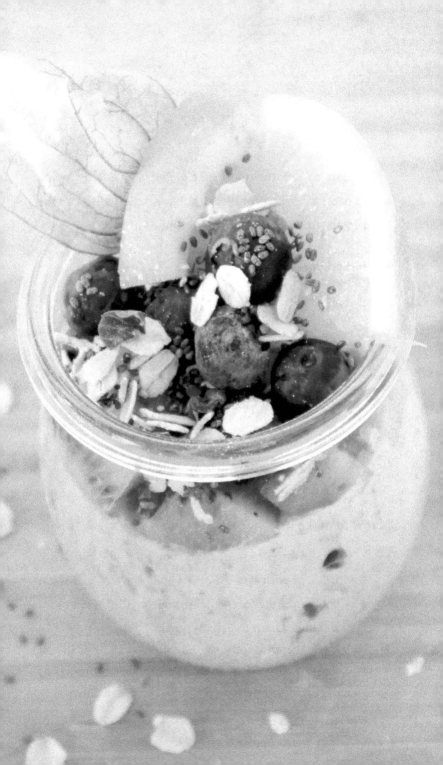

RECIPE #17: OATS WITH FRUITY GOODS AND ALMOND MILK

Breakfast or an afternoon snack – why not? This recipe with oats, cherries, plums and nuts, enriched with canna-milk will surely put you in a good mood.

What you need:

- 1/2 cup cannabis infused almond milk (see previous recipes)
- 1 cup of oats: keep your oats soaked in lemon juice – freshly squeezed
- 3 plums without pits and chopped
- 10 cherries without pits
- 1 tbsp. of pistachios – shelled
- 3 tbsp. of almonds – chopped and raw
- 5 Figs – dried and chopped

How to make it:

1. Drain the oats from the lemon juice and put them in a pot with two glasses of boiling water. Let them cook until they are al dente which will take 15 to 20 minutes. Drain the excess water.

2. Keep the stove on low heat and put the figs in the drained oats along with half a cup (or a bit more) of canna-milk. Stir and cook until the figs dissolve.

3. Pour into bowls and top with all the nuts and fruits from the list and enjoy!

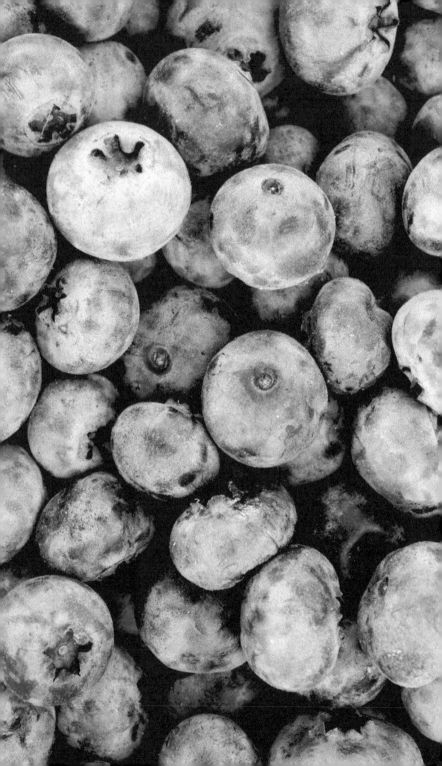

RECIPE #18: BLUEBERRY AND PEACH ALMOND MILK

If you are looking for a nutritious drink that can make a great choice for a liquid snack or refreshment, don't miss out on trying blueberry and peach canna-milk.

What you need:

- 1 cup of cannabis infused almond milk
- ½ cup of blueberries – frozen
- ½ cup of peach – frozen and sliced
- ½ teaspoon of vanilla extract
- ½ cup of oats
- 1 tbsp. of maple syrup or brown rice syrup

How to make it:

1. You are just one step away from this liquid delight. The only thing you need to is put syrup, fruits, oats, vanilla extract and canna-milk in blender or food processor and pulse until you get a smooth liquid.
2. Pour into a glass and enjoy!

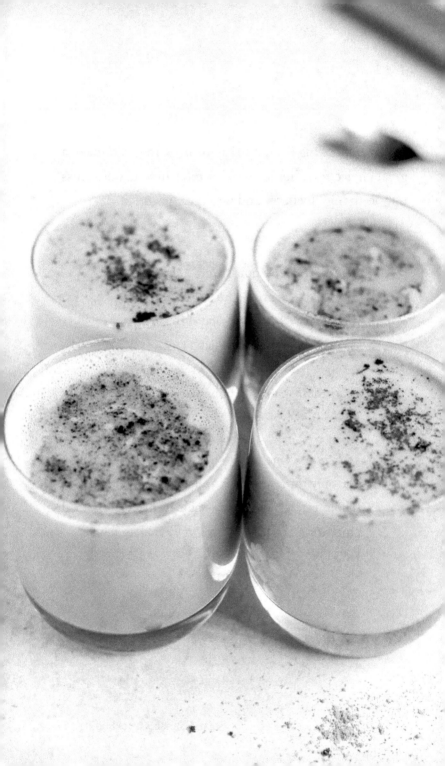

Recipe #19: Strawberry Canna-Milk Smoothie

We are saving refreshments in form of canna-milk drinks for the end, so brace yourself and try tofu and strawberry smoothie with canna-milk.

What you need:

- 10 strawberries – whole and frozen
- 1 cup of cannabis infused almond milk
  (see previous recipes)
- 2 tbsp. of sugar - organic

How to make it:

The only thing you need to take care of before preparing drinks is to have canna-milk ready just before trying our canna-smoothies or a couple of days before. Make sure cannabis used for making canna-milk has gone through decarboxylation process.

1. Put the strawberries, canna-milk and sugar in a blender or a food processor and blend until you get a smooth liquid.
2. Pour into a glass and enjoy your cool drink.

Recipe #20: Acai and Cherry Almond Milk Smoothie

And last, but not least: a wonderful smoothie made from power berry acai, cherries and canna-milk.

What you need:

- ½ cup of cannabis infused almond milk (see previous recipes)
- 3 ½ oz. of acai fruit puree – frozen and sugar-free
- ½ cup of cherries – frozen and without pits
- 1 tbsp. of almond butter
- 2 tsp. of brown rice syrup or maple syrup

How to make it:

1. Put the acai frozen puree, cherries, maple or brown rice syrup, almond butter and canna-milk in the blender. Pulse until you have a smooth liquid.
2. Pour into a glass and enjoy the fabulous effects of canna-milk and acai combined with the syrup sweetness and mild sourness of cherries.

RECIPE #21: MARY JANE'S MARIJUANA TEA

This tea has more of a "chill" vibe to it, delicious way to medicate and fly!

What you need:

- 1 Bag of tea per person
- 1 teaspoon of cannabis coconut oil per person

How to make it:

1. Add the 1 tsp. of cannabis coconut oil and a tea bag to a cup.
2. Boil the water and pour it in.
3. Let the cannabis coconut oil fully dissolve.
4. Remove the tea bag, add milk if you like it, and consume

Pro tip: Add mint, cinnamon, ginger, lemon and other tasty things to your liking. Try a pinch of black pepper; it might sound weird but it's a personal favorite.

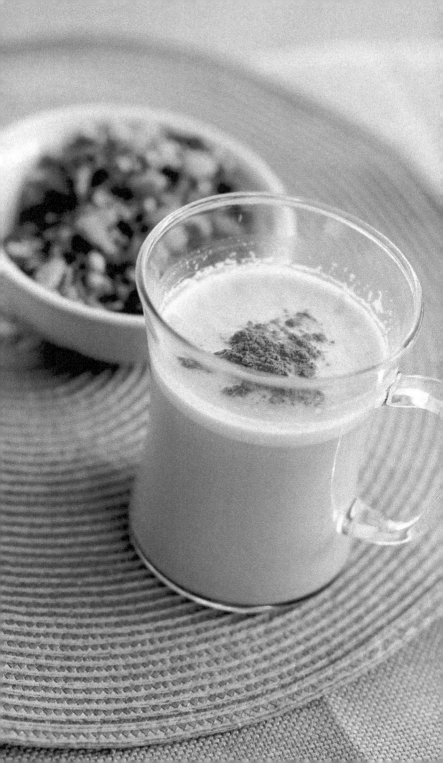

Recipe #22: Cannabis Chai

Spicy and sweet, a favorite recipe for cold and warm days, this works all the time!

What you need:

- 2 tsp. potent cannabis coconut oil
- ¾ cup pre-made tea of your choice (lemon is recommended)
- 2 cups water
- 4 cups almond milk (can be infused)
- ¼ cup sugar
- 1inch cinnamon stick
- 6 cloves
- 6 green cardamom pods, cracked
- 6 black peppercorns
- 1 tsp. fresh minced ginger
- ¼ cup half-and-half cream

How to make it:

1. Put the cannabis oil, water, almond milk, sugar, cinnamon, cloves, cardamom, peppercorns and ginger in a pan and bring to a boil.
2. Once boiling, lower the flame and let simmer for 15-20 minutes or until the Bhang becomes really fine and blended well.

3. Let it cool, strain the mixture with a cheese cloth into a jar, and keep it covered.

4. Pour ¼ cup of half-and-half cream and ¾ cup of strained tea in a cup. Heat it in the microwave and serve.

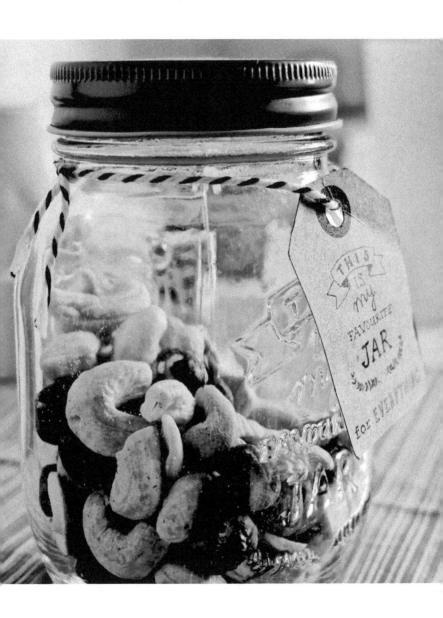

Recipe #23: Cannabis Granola

What you need:

- 1½ cups rolled oats
- ¼ cup chopped walnuts
- ¼ cup shredded unsweetened coconut
- 2 tbsp. dried chopped cherries
- 2 tbsp. whole flaxseed
- 2 tbsp. cannabis coconut oil
- 2 tbsp. honey
- ½ tsp. ground cinnamon

How to make it:

1. Preheat the oven to 300F.
2. Put all the ingredients in a large bowl and toss together well. Taste and add more maple syrup or cinnamon, if desired.
3. Spread the granola in one layer on a rimmed baking sheet.
4. Bake your granola, stirring every 10 minutes, until golden brown, about 30 minutes.
5. Let the granola cool on the baking sheet; it will be soft when it first comes out of the oven but will crisp up as it cools.

RECIPE #24: NO BAKE FUDGE

Be careful with dosing as this recipe can be extremely potent due to the large amount of infused coconut oil.

What you need:

- 2 lbs. / 7 cups of powdered sugar
- 1 cup of cocoa powder
- 1 lb. cannabis coconut oil
- 1 tsp. of vanilla essence
- 1 cup of peanut butter

How to make it:

1. Melt the infused coconut oil and peanut butter in a saucepan or double boiler and add the vanilla essence
2. In a large bowl, mix together the powdered sugar and cocoa.
3. Add the melted ingredients and mix well.
4. Press into a flat pan, and place in the fridge until firm.

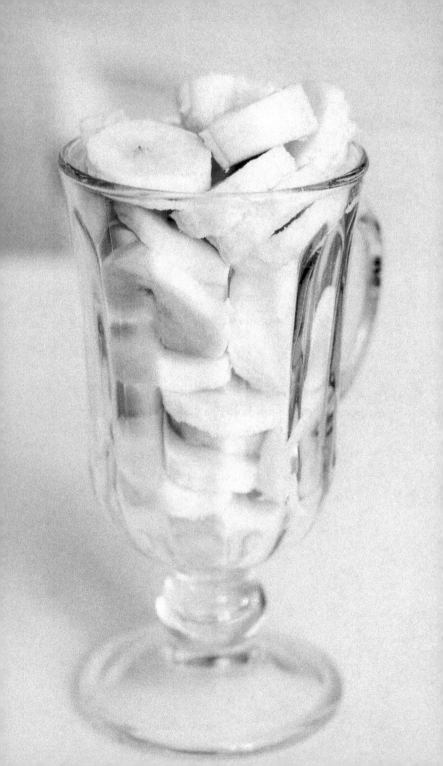

Recipe #25: Cannabanana-Peanut Butter Ice Cream

Best to serve cold while it is hot outside; be cautious, hot weather and edibles can turn you in to a sloth and too much will be quite uncomfortable.

What you need:

- 3 cups infused almond or coconut milk (½ of both is possible)
- ½ cup sugar
- 1 tbsp. corn starch
- Pinch of salt
- 4 bananas, pureed
- ½ cup peanut butter (optional)

How to make it:

1. Combine infused almond milk, coconut milk, sugar and corn-starch in a large saucepan and whisk together thoroughly. Cook over medium heat while stirring constantly until mixture starts to thicken, about 10 minutes. Remove from heat and allow to warm.
2. Pour the warm cannamilk mixture through a fine strainer and into a large bowl. Discard any solids.
3. Chill the cannamilk mixture uncovered in refrigerator for 1 hour; stir occasionally. Place plastic wrap on top

of milk mixture after 1 hour. Let chill for another 12 to 24 hours.

4. Pour cold mixture into 1½ quart ice cream freezer container and freeze.

5. Remove container from freezer after 2 hours, or until ice cream starts to firm but is still soft. Stir in banana puree and peanut butter with your spatula.

6. Mix well until peanut butter is equally distributed.

7. Return the container to freezer for another 6 hours, or until ice cream is firm.

8. Let it stand at room temperature for 5 minutes before serving.

Pro tip: Drizzle some jelly on top of your ice-cream to get some of that Peanut Butter Jelly Cannabanana action going and enjoy this epic combination! For super charge: add some extra cannamilk; mix it up in to a milk shake and have all the boys chilling in your yard!

RECIPE #26: MARY'S BERRIES SHERBET

What you need:

- 5 cups fresh blackberries
- 2 cups sugar
- 2 ½ cups infused coconut milk
- 1 tbsp. lemon juice

How to make it:

1. Blend blackberries and sugar together in food processor until smooth.
2. Pour the pureed berries through strainer and into a bowl. Discard seeds.
3. Mix the coconut milk into the blackberry puree. Stir in lemon juice.
4. Pour berry/milk mixture into an ice cream freezer container; freeze for 3 hours.
5. Let stand at room temperature for 5 minutes before serving.

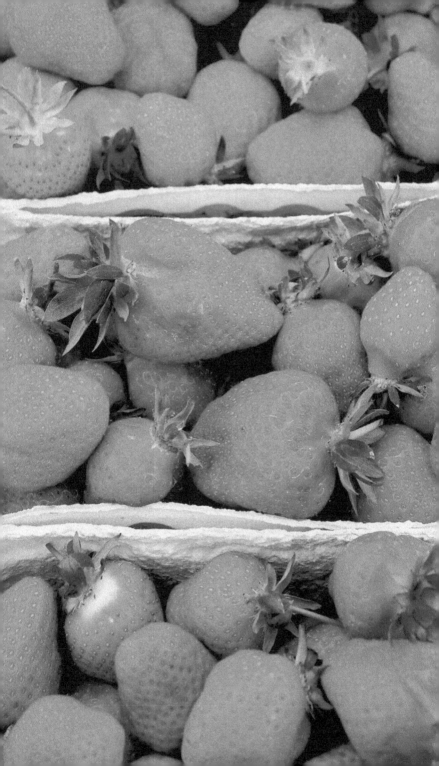

RECIPE #27: MARY-JANE'S STRAWBERRIES

What you need:

- 1 ½ cups dark chocolate chips (vegan)
- ¼ cup cannabis coconut oil
- 20 strawberries (with stems)
- ¼ cup vegan sprinkles

How to make it:

- Heat dark chocolate and cannabis coconut oil in a microwave safe bowl. Remove and stir every 20 seconds until melted.
- Dip dry strawberries in chocolate one at a time, allowing excess chocolate to drip back into bowl.
- Dip the tips of each chocolate coated strawberry into the blue sprinkles.
- Sit strawberries on wax lined plate to dry.
- Chill strawberries in fridge 20 minutes before serving.

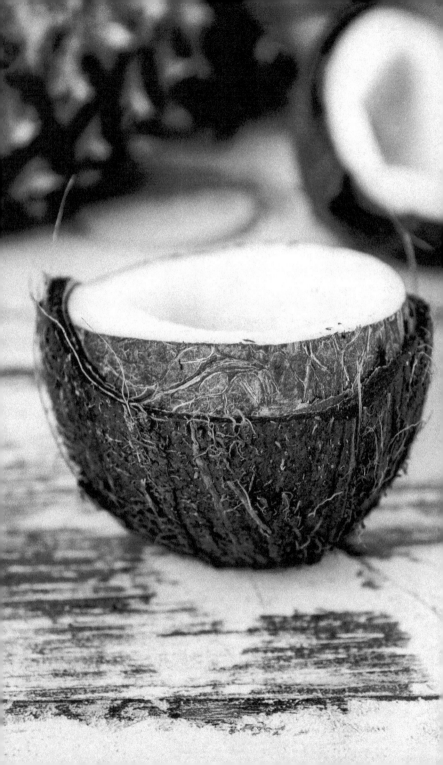

RECIPE #28: COCONUT BERRY BOMBS

What you need:

- 1 cup coconut butter
- 1 cup cannabis coconut oil
- ½ cup fresh or frozen fruit of your choice (raspberries, blackberries, blueberries, etc.)
- ½ tsp. sweetener of your choice (for example: 3 drops of stevia)
- ¼ tsp. vanilla powder
- 1 tbsp. lemon juice

How to make it:

1. Place coconut oil, coconut butter and fruit (only if you chose frozen fruit) in a pot and heat on stove.
2. Mix thoroughly, then let cool.
3. Place mixture in a blender.
4. Add remaining ingredients to blender.
5. Blend until smooth.
6. Spread mix on a pan lined with parchment paper. Spread evenly.
7. Place in refrigerator for about an hour or until cold and firm.
8. Once cold, cut into about 16 squares and put back into refrigerator.

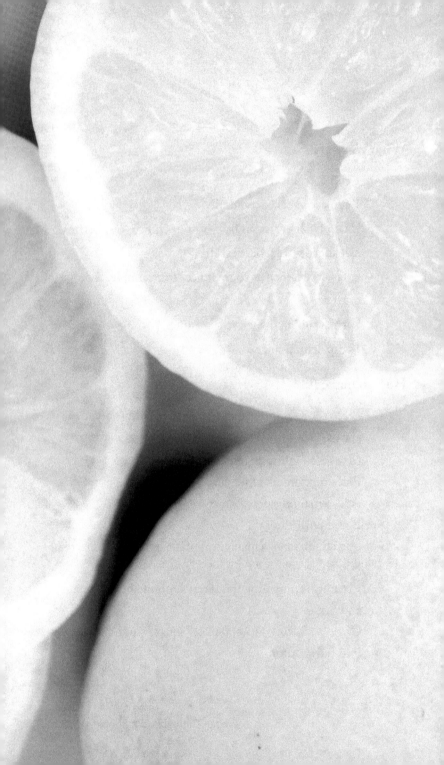

RECIPE #29: LEMON ZEST FAT BOMBS

What you need:

- ½ cup coconut butter (also sold in stores as creamed coconut, NOT coconut milk)
- ¼ cup cannabis coconut oil, softened
- lemon zest, finely grated from 1-2 lemons
- 3 drops of stevia
- 1 pinch of salt

How to make it:

1. Mix together all the ingredients, ensuring even mixing.
2. Fill mini cupcake molds with 1 tablespoon of the mixture.
3. Place tray in fridge for about an hour or until firm.

RECIPE #30: WALNUT CHOCOLATE BARS

What you need:

- ½ cup cannabis coconut oil (melted)
- 4 tbsp. cocoa powder
- 1 tbsp. sugar (or sweetener of your choice)
- 2 tbsp. tahini paste
- ¼ cup halved walnuts

How to make it:

1. Place all the ingredients except the walnuts in a pot on low heat.
2. Stir constantly until melted.
3. Let cool.
4. Pour mixture into molds (or ice trays) and place in refrigerator.
5. Once bars are almost firm, add a halved walnut on top of each bar and continue to refrigerate.

RECIPE #31: PEANUT BUTTER PECAN BARS

What you need:

- ½ cup peanut butter
- ½ cup cannabis coconut oil
- 1 tsp. vanilla extract
- 1 tbsp. vanilla syrup
- 1 cup pecans

How to make it:

1. Place coconut oil and peanut butter in a bowl and mix.
2. Warm mixture in a microwave for 30 seconds, then take out and mix some more.
3. Place mixture back in microwave for another 30 seconds. Repeat process until mixture is smooth.
4. Add extract, syrup and pecans and stir until well blended.
5. Separate mix into 4 separate rectangular molds to give thin, rectangular bar shape.
6. Place bars in refrigerator and let cool until firm.

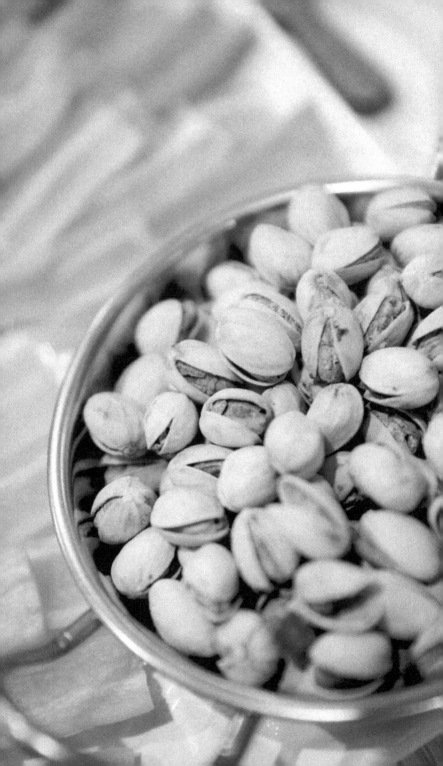

RECIPE #32: CHOCOLATE ORANGE NUT CLUSTERS

What you need:

- ½ cup pure dark cocoa powder
- ¼ cup cannabis coconut oil
- 1 ⅓ cups walnuts, chopped
  (or any nut of your preference)
- 1 tsp. cinnamon
- ½ tbsp. orange zest (finely grated)

How to make it:

1. Place dark chocolate along with a bit of water in a pot.
2. Stir on low heat.
3. Add coconut oil, orange zest, chopped walnuts and cinnamon and stir well.
4. Spoon about one tablespoon of the mixture into mini candy parchment cups.
5. Refrigerate overnight.

Recipe #33: Vanilla Bombs

What you need:

- 1 cup macadamia nuts
- ½ cup cannabis coconut oil
- 2 tsp. vanilla extract

How to make it:

1. Place all ingredients in a blender and blend until smooth.
2. Pour mixture into an ice tray and place in fridge until firm.

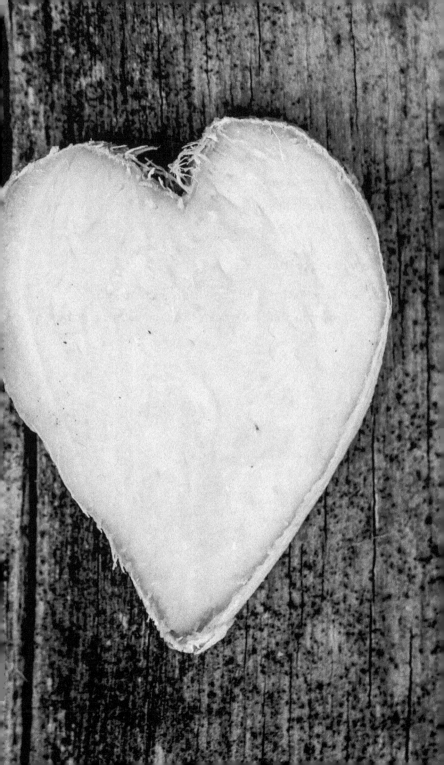

Recipe #34: Ginger Fat Bombs

What you need:

- ⅓ cup coconut butter
- ⅓ cup cannabis coconut oil
- ¼ cup shredded coconut, unsweetened
- 1 tsp. ginger powder

How to make it:

1. In a bowl, mix all ingredients until smooth.
2. Pour mixture into molds (for example, ice cube trays).
3. Place in fridge to set.

RECIPE #35: MINT CHOCOLATE FUDGE

What you need:

- 1½ cups cannabis coconut oil, melted
- 1¼ cups almond butter (or nut butter of choice)
- ½ cup favorite natural sugar or sweetener (all work just fine)
- ½ cup dried parsley flakes (crazy, right?!)
- 2 tsp. vanilla extract
- 1 tsp. peppermint extract
- 1 pinch of salt
- 10 oz. melted dark chocolate (optional, again use store bought)

How to make it:

1. Add all ingredients in a blender. Blend till smooth.
2. Pour into a non-stick pan and freeze until firm.
3. If adding chocolate, drizzle on top once the fudge is firm.
4. Keep refrigerated.

FREE BONUS

Don't forget to grab your copy of 'Cannabis 101: A Short Introduction To Growing Medical Marijuana With Our Favorite Strains And Recipes For Cannabis Infused Cooking'.

Subscribe to our newsletter by using this link:

http://happyhealthygreen.life/cannabis-newsletter

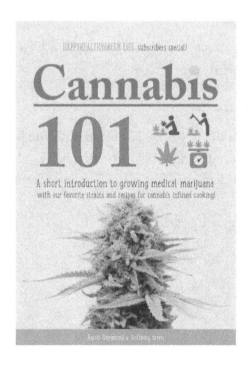

By subscribing to our newsletter, you will receive cannabis infused recipes, the best medical and recreational marijuana tips and even more free eBooks right in your inbox.

We also offer you a unique opportunity to read future vegan cookbooks for absolutely free...

Get your hands on awesome tips, recipes and instant access to 'Cannabis 101'. Subscribe to the cannabis newsletter and grab your copy at:

http://happyhealthygreen.life/cannabis-newsletter

Enter your email address to get instant access.

* We don't like spam and understand you don't like spam either. We'll email you no more than 2 times per week.*

THANK YOU

Finally, if you enjoyed this book, then we would like to ask you for a small favor. Would you be kind enough to leave an honest review for this book? It'd be greatly appreciated by both the future reader and me!

You can send us your feedback on Amazon.

Did you discover any grammar mistakes, confusing explanations or wrongful information? Don't hesitate to send us an email!
You can reach us at **info@happyhealthygreen.life**

We promise to get back to you as soon as time allows us. If this book requires a revision, we'll send you the updated eBook for free after the revised book is available.

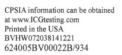

9 789492 788108